HOME REMEDIES FOR HEART DISEASE PREVENTION

Scientifically Proven Based on Healthy LifeStyles.

Sheldon Feil

Table of Contents

Introduction

As one of the leading causes of death and hospitalization in both men and women in nearly all countries in America, Europe, and Asia as well as in many other parts of the world, heart disease represents a significant public health threat or burden. Surveillance is still the most effective tool for evaluating the burden of disease, assessing its growing trend, planning preventive actions at both the population and individual levels, and estimating the efficacy of prevention, despite the pressing need to implement comprehensive strategies to address this growing epidemic in the

United States. In the United States, the most common heart diseases are those caused by atherosclerosis, primarily ischemic heart disease (IHD) and stroke. Heart disease clinically manifests itself in middle age and later in life, after many years of exposure to unhealthy lifestyles (such as an unhealthy diet, physical inactivity, and a smoking habit) and risk factors (such as a family history of heart disease) (high blood pressure, high cholesterolemia, diabetes, obesity etcetera).

Even though it is extremely common, its occurrence is largely preventable, making it a top priority for public health and environmental sustainability efforts. Clinical studies have shown that cardiovascular risk can be reversible,' meaning that by lowering the level of risk factors, it is possible to reduce the number and severity of events or delay the occurrence of events altogether. Even though heart disease has a predominantly acute clinical onset, it often progresses slowly, resulting in a significant loss of quality of life, disability, and a lifelong reliance on healthcare services and medications. In the long run, this will result in premature death as well as adverse outcomes in elderly people such as cognitive impairment, dementia, and decreased physical performance. Dietary cholesterol is associated with significant societal costs, which include not only those directly associated with health care and social services but also those associated with illness benefits and retirement, the impact on families and caregivers, as well as the loss of years of productive life.

Types of Heart Disease

- Coronary artery disease (CAD): This has been the most common symptom of a cardiovascular problem (CAD). Carotid artery disease (CAD) is a condition characterized by the formation of blockages in the coronary arteries, which are the vessels that supply blood to the heart. As a result, the circulation to your heart muscle may be reduced, preventing it from receiving the oxygen that it needs to function properly. It is important to note that atherosclerosis, also known as arterial hardening, is a condition that typically occurs before the onset of the disease. Heart disease, also known as sinus tachycardia, can cause breathing difficulties.

- Arrhythmias of the heart: Your heart beats in an irregular pattern when you have an arrhythmia. Serious arrhythmias are most commonly caused by other heart problems, but they can also occur on their own.

- Heart Failure: Heart failure occurs when your heart does not pump blood as efficiently as it should to meet the demands of your body. It is usually caused by coronary artery disease, but it can also occur as a result of other conditions such as thyroid disease, high blood pressure, heart muscle disease (cardiomyopathy), or certain other diseases and conditions.

•   Heart Valve Disease: The four chambers of your heart, the lungs, and blood vessels are all connected by four valves that open and close to direct blood flow between the chambers. An abnormality may make it difficult for a valve to open and close properly. When this occurs, your blood flow may be obstructed, or blood may leak from your body. It is possible that your valve will not open and close properly.

•   Pericardial   Disease: Virus infection, inflammatory diseases such as lupus or rheumatoid arthritis, or an injury to your pericardium are the most common causes of pericarditis. Pericarditis is a common complication of open-heart surgery.

•   Cardiomyopathy:

Cardiomyopathy, also known as pericarditis, is a disease of the heart tissue or cardiac muscle. It becomes strained, thickened, or stiff as a result of this. Your heart may become too weak to pump effectively.

Risk Factors for Heart Disease Development

•   Age: Growing aged increases your chances of developing damaged and narrowed arteries, as well as a weaker or thick heart, among other things. Growing aged increases your chances of developing damaged and narrowed arteries, as well as a weaker or thick heart, among other things.

•	Gender: Men are more at risk of developing heart disease than women. After menopause, women are at increased risk of developing breast cancer.

•	Ancestors and forefathers: You are more likely to develop coronary artery disease if your family has a history of heart disease, particularly if one of your parents had it at a young age.

- Smoking. Carbon monoxide can damage the inner lining of your blood vessels, making them more susceptible to atherosclerosis. Nicotine tightens your blood vessels. Tobacco users are more likely than non-tobacco users to suffer an injury.

- Poor diet. Having a diet that is high in fat, salt, sugar, and cholesterol can increase your risk of developing heart disease.

- High blood pressure: In the absence of treatment, unchecked high blood pressure can lead to toughening and hypertrophy of the artery walls, which can restrict the pathways through which blood flows. A lack of control over one's blood pressure can result in the coarsening and hypertrophy of one's artery walls, which can narrow the passageways through which blood can flow and cause death.

• High levels of cholesterol in the blood: High levels of cholesterol in your blood can increase the risk of plaque formation and atherosclerosis.

• Diabetes. Diabetes increases the likelihood of developing heart disease. Obesity and high blood pressure are two risk factors that are shared by both conditions.

- Obesity. Weight gain is usually associated with a rapid deterioration of other heart disease risk factors

- Inactivity on a physical level: Lack of physical activity is also linked to many types of heart disease, as well as some of the other risk factors associated with it.

- Stress. Stress that is not relieved can damage your arteries and exacerbate other heart problems.

- Poor dental health. It is critical to brush and floss your teeth and gums regularly, as well as to have regular dental checkups. Endocarditis is a condition that occurs when bacteria enter the bloodstream and travel to the heart. It is caused by poor oral hygiene and decayed teeth and gums.

Potential problems of Heart Disease

•	Heart failure. When your heart is unable to pump enough blood to meet your body's needs, you can develop heart failure, a common rare condition of heart disease. Congenital heart defects, cardiovascular disease, valvular heart disease, infections of the heart, and cardiomyopathy are all examples of conditions that can cause heart failure.

•	Heart attack. A cardiac arrest is caused by a blood clot that prevents blood from flowing through a blood vessel that supplies the heart, potentially damaging or destroying a portion of the cardiac muscle. Cardiovascular disease such as atherosclerosis is a risk factor for heart attacks.

• Stroke. The risk factors for cardiovascular disease can also lead to an ischemic stroke, which occurs when the arteries leading to your brain narrow or block, allowing insufficient blood to reach your brain. Because brain tissue begins to die within minutes of a stroke, it is considered a medical emergency.

- Aneurysm. An aneurysm is a bulge in the wall of your artery and is a serious complication that can occur anywhere in your body. If an aneurysm ruptures, you could suffer from life-threatening internal bleeding.

- Peripheral artery disease. When you have peripheral artery disease, blood flow to your extremities, usually your legs, is reduced. This causes symptoms, the most notable of which is leg pain when walking (claudication). Atherosclerosis can also cause peripheral artery disease.

- Sudden cardiac arrest. An arrhythmia is a sudden, unexplained cessation of heart function, breathing, and consciousness. Sudden cardiac arrest is a life-threatening situation. It can lead to sudden cardiac death if not treated promptly.

Ways to Prevent Heart Disease

1.   Avoiding Smoking

Stopping smoking or using smokeless tobacco is one of the best things you can do for your heart. Even if you don't smoke, you should avoid being around people who are.

2.   Get up and move around for at least 30-60 minutes each day.

The risk of heart disease can be reduced by regular, daily physical activity. Losing weight is easier when you're physically active. It also lowers the risk of developing other heart-stressing conditions, such as hypertension.

3. Eat a heart-healthy diet

Protecting the heart, lowering blood pressure and cholesterol, and reducing the risk of type 2 diabetes are all benefits of a healthy diet. The following foods are included in a heart-healthy diet:

- Fruits and veg

- a legume.

- Eat lean meats and fish.

- Dairy foods that are low in fat or fat-free

- a complete food

- Olive oil, for example, is a good source of healthy fats.

Examples of heart-healthy diets include the Mediterranean diet and the Dietary Approach to Stop Hypertension (DASH) plan.

Limit the following:

- Processed carbohydrates

- Sugar

- Alcohol

- Salt

- Saturated fat (found in red meat and full-fat dairy products) and trans fat (found in fried fast food, chips, and baked goods)Saturated fat and trans fat (found in red meat and whole milk) (found in fried fast food, chips, and baked goods)

4. Maintaining a healthy weight is essential.

Heart disease is more likely to occur if you are obese, particularly around the middle of your body. High blood pressure, high cholesterol, and type 2 diabetes are all made more likely by being overweight or obese.

5. Ensure that you get a good night's sleep

The majority of adults require at least seven hours of sleep per night. Don't put off getting enough sleep. To get the best night's sleep, stick to a regular bedtime and wake-up time. Make it easier to fall asleep by keeping your bedroom dark and quiet.

6. Manage your feelings of stress.

Overeating, binge drinking, or smoking are all unhealthy ways for some people to cope with stress. Improve your health by finding healthier ways to cope with stress.

Examples include regular exercise, relaxation techniques, and meditation.

7. Maintaining a healthy lifestyle requires regular health screenings.

Heart and blood vessels can be damaged by hypertension and elevated cholesterol. However, if you don't get tested for these conditions, you may never know if you have them. Regular screening can tell you what your numbers are and if you need to do something about them.

• The systolic Blood Pressure: In most cases, blood pressure screenings begin at a young age. Heart disease and stroke are two of the leading killers in the United States, and high blood pressure is a risk factor for both of these diseases.

• Cholesterol levels in the bloodstream: Adults' cholesterol levels are typically checked every four to six years at the very least. There are certain risk factors, such as a family history of heart disease, that necessitate cholesterol screening earlier than the usual age of 20.

• detecting and treating diabetes type 2: Heart disease is linked to diabetes. Early screening for diabetes may be recommended if you have risk factors such as being overweight or having a family history of the disease. Screening begins at 45, and retesting is recommended every three years after that.

Medicines and lifestyle changes may be prescribed by your doctor if you have a medical condition like high cholesterol, high blood pressure, or diabetes. Make sure to follow your doctor's instructions for taking your medication and adopting a healthy lifestyle.